Invisible Medicine

Thomas Medonis

The Healing of
the Earth

Thomas Medonis

An essence known as ether has hitherto existed. This immeasurable substance isn't wildly known to the populace. This etheric ocean that fills the space throughout our universe is transmitting electronic currents into your very own etheric body this very second, a body that is composed of energy threads. A contemporary definition of ether is that two organic groups attach to an oxygen atom. Minerals attached to oxygen atoms will therefore conduct energy currents. Are we a formation of wires?

How can electricity flow through the air?

Ancient philosophy claimed that ether was the medium that filled space. Through the study and practice of ancient spiritual wisdom one can obtain a super sensibility toward the spiritual world that forms the ether. The pervasive imperceptible spirits throughout nature that form our earth can become visible. The mind must, however, perform a transmutation in order to develop this spiritual sense. Think of the fine roots of a plant "magnetizing in" all the essential elements within the soil for its developing form. If one is to pursue the consuming desires of form (ego), then no super-sensibility can occur. We must be reborn to join the kingdom.

A soul center dwells in every living form and emits a soul body. The soul is omnipresent and omnipotent. An indefinable essence at the root of our very existence is the mystery that makes humans what they are (I will later make the same case for the sun). A metaphor can be drawn here: that the souls evolution exists like that of the force within a seed. Soul is not the matter presented in seed form, but rather the force that will extract the living being out of the seed to fulfill its purpose in physical manifestation.

Modern physics has proven the existence of these eternal elements and their emitting rays. The proof for perpetual life on this earth is located right within the essence of every being. Everyone has soul. It all depends how far from soul awareness each individual is. The invisible force that animates the body is one of the three main bodies which form mans physique, the physical body and the eternal soul being the other two.

In other words, without certain invisible omnipresent forces man could not exist in the physical form. No living being could. The great separation between man and animal, who both house soul, is the great power conducted by the higher mind. It actually takes more energy to generate thought, than perform feats of physical labor. Think about that.

Where is your energy heading, while concentrating on one particular issue? Over or under stimulation of vital energy centers brings about disorder in the concentrated energy core. Disease thus unravels through the central nervous system, the endocrine system: the great system that transmits emotional energy into the blood (Blood boiling, cold blooded, etc.)

Mind, body, and soul of man are linked by these supersensible connections. These energy centers harmonize the flow of blood. Emotions serve as the catalyst for humans' evolution, as sense perception has formed man through the ego's design.

This is why emotion will always exist on a certain frequency of conscientiousness. Thoughts are therefore connected with our own organs. Organs are connected to glands and the glands are run by the energy center (chakra). This is a way of linking certain disorders with certain energy centers. Thus if there is over or under activity of a center, conflict and deformity will ensue.

There are seven main energy centers within a human's etheric and physical structure. These focal points serve as hubs for emotional/spiritual vibrations. They are all equally important for their distinct role. The expression of the soul would be deficient if an imbalance exists within a center.

I will begin by discussing the two lower centers. These lower centers are defined as the Base, or root, center and the Sacral center. The

Base center, chakra, is the central internal provider of absolute life. The Sacral center, chakra, too is imperative for health as it transmits the procreative desire nature, as well as the lower impulses brought on by the ego's carnal desires. This Sacral Center, conversely, has a great potency and can give birth to our spiritual re-awakening. Our needs are the results of varying impulses. The survival impulse originates in the root chakra. The motion of emotion within the physique also originates in these lower centers, as the animal impulse is constant.

Emotional attitudes toward the attainment of external gratification evolve over stages of development. Through these desire vibrations we produce, each soul expresses the illumination of its own soul/astral/karmic/etheric body-whatever you choose to call it. The physical develops with its soul's evolution.

Hitherto, our emotions have formed a desire body that is incorporated with both our etheric body and soul. Some would argue that a pleasure body is accompanied by a pain body.

When our astral/etheric body detaches from the physical body and enters into the astral plane, sensory skills no longer exist in this dimension. Pure emotion at certain elemental frequencies is all that now fuels the astral body at this stage of spiritual growth. Therefore, the desire/emotional/karmic body is formed through experience on earth in each lifetime. Disintegration of the emotional experience occurs in accordance with the soul's crystallization.

In a higher frequency the lower centers reach a spiritual sense of wholeness, completion. The lower the vibration the more we are geared toward our lower animal nature. That being said, the base of the spine, the seat of the lower self, is in close proximity with the procreative forces. Therefore, the indescribable super sensible impulses of the soul are corrupted when received by the animal ego. The emotional force is driven by the ego. How is one to transcend the temptations vibrating within the sacral center? Compromising with great forces within the physique, along with receiving external impulses appropriately, is a start- Meditate! The elimination of balanced energy conduction forms dysfunction in the harmony of the finer instruments, such as the nerves and organs. The organs within the jurisdiction of the disordered center are the first to alter.

Thus the mind holds the key! The animal instinct can mutate into a work of fine art. Disavowal of the self's cravings is the beginning of the end for misdirected energy. If the reader is able to accept the suggestion that the world does not revolve around the accomplishment of his/her wants and desires, then the bridge for a higher consciousness may be discovered. Rather the human body serves as a microcosm of the universe we live in- seven planets, seven centers. Each center therefore serves as a planet within the structure of man, with the result being proper magnetic pull and radiation. To understand the design of the etheric body one must understand the purpose of each center.

Some consider the center located in the gut the second brain, or it may be called the solar plexus center. This energy center forms the perception of self, in which a cycle of emotional impulses runs through this chakra. Any instant judgment is formed in the mind this center disrupts its equilibrium. To replenish this center the individual must begin to connect with their divine purpose- a purpose comparable to that of the Sun's etheric body. Some may argue the universal consciousness is still in this stage of recognition of soul.

Ironically, the center above the solar plexus is the heart center- The home for love. A center we must all begin to truly recognize and grasp. It is the one center that rhythmically retains the impulse of infinite unconditional love. There are many definitions for this one eternal trait that will's man to overcome great impassible obstacles. Thus true love is impossible as long as the heart center is disordered and begins to harden.

The throat center is the home of creative divinity. The bestowed wisdom of the higher invisible elemental rays is clearly evident through the higher consciousness of this center. Addiction is a result of dysfunction within this center, an argument that can be made for disorder in any of the center's. Thus, it may begin to become clear how the upper centers can be manipulated from their equilibrium in order to fill the soul's sensations presented to the ego. A misinterpretation of the soul's purpose unfolds externally. Thus if the soul's will is not performing in accordance with divine laws than the creative genius is not connected with divine thought. Creativity is performed for the ego. Thus for many, desires take charge and eliminate the soul's innovative desire to employ change in order to align the macro- soul with the micro-soul. Humanics in action!

Now with so much talk of soul-consciousness we will work up to the centers connected with the mind. The Ajna center sits right between the eyes and it is called the great source of intuition and imagination. The pineal gland's spiritual sense is the doorway into the etheric body.

The last center to mention is the crown center. The Crown is found around the very top of the head. The soul's antenna! But in order for this device to form and run properly- - a change of direction in thought must occur. If a change develops in support of natural growth and budding flowers, the mind will begin to receive the impulses from a higher consciousness. Subtle changes in thinking forms an imperceptible pervasive power that changes the way in which our mind collects impulses. Nothing stays constant in the Universe but the Absolute One, thoughts will forever flow through the ether. Thus a simple floating divine thought could ultimately drive an individual to transform his ego. A divine purpose only runs parallel with pure thoughts.

To surely remove ego the mind must separate three individual forces within the mind. Will, feeling, and thought must be untangled in order for man to find the center within his Ajna center.

If this center is recognized the human will soon discover electric currents running through the etheric body. Subtleties ignored in the past now appear as currents within the individual etheric mold. Once the separation is made between thought, feeling, and will in the mind, the next step is to separate the same principles, throughout the body. Therefore a more defined energy vibration begins to develop within the mind. The mind will begin to pay homage to the soul. This mindset will soon present the powerful innocence and reverence held by the infinite soul. Its omnipresence becomes a dominating constant. Thus a soul body illuminates around the etheric and physical vehicle.

Divine thought in the human mind is all manufactured by the invisible elements emitted through the suns invisible rays. Rays pushed forth by the great force of the energy manifestation within the sun are also available for human's benefit through a mental transmutation. We no longer are absorbing or releasing energy that hinders natural growth. Death and decay are qualities we recognize, but do not associate with. Rebirth, renewal, and springtime buds, are all qualities familiar to the spirit of natural well-being. Living with the seasons.

We are no longer a micro-planet, but now we too are a sun emitting rays to benefit the entirety of the universe, with not one thought for self. The increasing vision of natural growth within the permanence of the all-pervading etheric rays will always attract my devotion.

It is true- the mental and chemical pollution we emit is purified by the suns rays and various dimensions. As we relinquish the poisonous toxins through various means (breathing, sweating), the particle matter performs a metamorphous. The physical body is forever developing. The etheric and soul body also undergo changes- with greatest of intensity at the time of death. Truly, death is a time we should most celebrate. It is the soul's return ascent home, shedding the Astral body along the journey.

Our individual Astral body is a microcosm of the greater universal Astral Plane, which some would define as the Ether. Even in physical death, our invisible bodies survive in this Astral Plane. The astral body, following death, begins to call the Astral Plane home. Yes, spirits live within the seven main elements that compose the ether. These seven elements are also widely known as the seven rays.

Spirits and living impulses survive within the elemental ray they are attracted to- The Law of

Attraction. There is no equilibrium or neutral within this Astral Plane- high or low, angry or sad. With the mineral content existing in the ether, the connection is made in the physical body with these forces through the magnetic pull of our mind's impulses.

Again, disorder occurs in whichever of the centers that is over-stimulated at the time of thought. Thus we live with and breathe in the invisible dead astral thought carcasses of the past. One thing must be expressed again, there are good and bad rays that are received. It all must be balanced. The nature of the etheric elemental ray absorbed is therefore attracted by the cyclical mental activity.

A ray therefore becomes improper as its frequency enters a realm in which it doesn't connect. In order to grasp the nature of the seven rays we must first grasp all of their qualities. Qualities we can trace back to the sun's form. The rays reflect the seven fulfillments from the "seven Spirits before the throne of God"[i].

The sun is not an elemental ray, but what forms its cosmic force and emitting energies is all the result of the seven elemental God rays. With acceptance that the sun's rays are driven by seven essential rays, we can begin to understand the absolute reality. Through the cycle of time the space has hitherto filled with cosmic rays that develop universal logic, as well as the rays that promote the physical vegetable and animal kingdoms.

Thus the invisible force of the absolute one manifests into

concrete external form. This force is active in every life form, even in the invisible nature spirits that make up Earth's etheric body. This being said, there is a great difference between human and animal nature (at times). Humans have the ability to advance their mind, animals, more or less, are stuck in their station. Hence, higher knowledge is continually available in order to develop the mind into an instrument comparable to no other. It is, however, all in the individual's hands to decide whether to follow their own divine purpose or not.

It is the transmitting impulses from the emitting rays in the astral plane which structure vast traits. Research into the rays' powers would be an infinite task no doubt. The first three rays I will define, by legendary Alice A. Bailey, are "The Great Rays of Aspect". She believed consciousness could be separated into three individual categories by these three rays. The ray emitting red conducts the impulse of will and power. The blue ray emits love and emotions. The yellow ray emits intelligence in thought.

These three supersensible rays bridge the gap between the concrete mind and the logic of the gods. These attributes are also necessary for the destiny of the present. All rays are constantly aligned to serve their divine purpose. We must connect! The next four rays will also be described through the color they emit.

These rays are considered those of "attribute". For one developed in color sensory, I have read somewhere that the lighter the shade envisioned the calmer the potency. The rays have polarizing effects.

The orange ray is considered the ray of harmony through conflict. The green rays emit the knowledge of science and concrete physical fact. The purple ray emits devotion and idealism into an energy center. The concluding indigo ray provides the impulse for order and ceremonial magic. Thus, these rays influence energy centers through the energy within the astral plane.

Within the Astral plane, four branches of nature have unraveled through this spirit of the cosmic rays. The mineral kingdom, the vegetable kingdom, the animal kingdom, and the human kingdom all could somewhat define the evolution of nature.

The mineral kingdom deserves essential praise for our development because of the extremes of static activity produced from mineral form-lifeless nature, on one side of the spectrum, and intensity of radiation on the other.

Radioactivity results from the mineral attachment to the atomic ether.

Next, the vegetable kingdom is grounded within the soil of the earth. We must keep in mind that whatever composes the soil, will compose the plant. This kingdom may provide a prime example of disorder within an energy center. Is the food you're eating natural?

Are man's acts driven by materialistic cravings depleting the equilibrium of the earth's purpose?

Thirdly, the animal kingdom, just as all kingdoms, is ever evolving. The development of instinct and intuition enable man to be the king of this category. It is in his liberation from this lower self that man will promote himself into the human kingdom.

The human kingdom we could still consider undeveloped as it has not fully emerged. This is the kingdom where the higher elements connect with the device in the head that only could become developed through divine intent. "What stands above, sits below." Thus liberation from the thoughts triggered by external forms allow one to begin to understand the emotional energy fueling the macrocosm.

The mind's development is similar as to that which unfolds within the mineral kingdom. The depths and dimensions reached during the crystallization of a mineral also unfold within man's mind. Hence, if one develops the mind to such a fine gold impulse, one will emit a golden aura. Is this mind transmutation already determined within the evolutionary rings of the universe? Or is it a race against time to repair our destruction?

There are evolutionary stages within the life cycle of a mineral, in which their forms could be divided into three sections- baser metals, standard metals, and semiprecious stones. Now what if human activity is altering the mineral structure of the ether?

Is manmade particle matter disrupting the ether provided by the heavens? Is there too much pollution for the rays to purify? Are the rays so severely polluted that our individual etheric centers are dysfunctioning as a result?

Destruction of nature may reflect the same deadly destructive power capable of removing our etheric form from our physical. Thus, it is of my greatest interest if it is possible for earth's physical form to break from its etheric body, just as a dying carcass breaks ties with the etheric and soul body. Is the earth withstanding such a great destructive disorder?

Some argue that humans have created the condition of the Earth. What if the fate of the world now lies in our hands. We continually drain the recourses out of the earth. Can the earth sustain itself through such rapid depletion? We are also adding tons of waste into the earth as well. Maybe we can passionately change all this. All we have done is take, take, take, we never have given back. The Earth needs a whole lot of unconditional love! What if it is possible to strengthen the earth. What if I told you microscopic bugs may be our solution. Micro-organisms are essential to soil composition and health. There are little parasites dancing around your body as you read.

Soil depletion is a great ill cast upon the earth. *Indefinable Spirits* live in the earth, in the plant, in the evaporating water, in the gases, in the air, in the heavens, all of which are essential to plant and human growth. What if those spirits are vastly depleted? Can they be restored?

Soil replenishment is where we should maybe begin to look-improved consistency. The extraction and absorption of cosmic, solar, and earthly forces at a greater magnetic attraction may portray the ability to rejuvenate and repair our earth. It must all be driven by spiritual ego nevertheless. This Divine Will for change can repair our de-energized food and repair ourselves within.

The most important thing I hope the reader takes from this work is that it is possible to fix yourself by first simply examining your soul. A simple task of correcting the flow of the spirit is a beginning. Sound health therefore develops in the mind rather than the physique. Now if the energies begin to change flow in order to repair our individual disorders, then maybe the energetic dysfunction we feed the ether will subside.

Some consider a portion of the natural spirits as ever changing microscopic parasites. This ever changing form is a clear indication as to why brain matter evolves. In "What is Biodynamics", Rudolf Steiner claims, "The human brain is the evolved product of elimination." What if there is no longer any beneficial natural spirits in our food? In a sense our food is depleted of nutrition to appease capital gain. What is a fruits value? The value of a fruit should not rest in its material impression, but rather in the composition of the elements that formed the material. There is a certain vitality in play that is necessary for both spiritual and plant growth.

It seems to me that vast unlimited energies have been spent on the analysis of a disease. What about the cure? Rather than make the effect the focal point, why not investigate and study the individual, as that, an individual. The causes and symptoms need to be traced back to its energy provider.

In conclusion, if there's a will, there's a way! We can accomplish anything, but we must first change within. We must unite ourselves with what is truly living, seen or unseen. It is now time to promote both the individual and universal well-being! Earth is in the process of dying, we need to heal it, and heal it now! Remember, soil with humus like substances in the process of decomposition contains living ether, and it is the soil that ultimately becomes the plant's mask.

Think of how we feed the earth in so many negative ways, non-disposable garbage, synthetics, dead carcasses filled with disease, water-soluble fertilizers. Yes, have you ever thought of the earth filled with dead decaying diseased carcasses? Cremation serves so many wonderful purposes. It keeps a body from taking up a nice sized plot. Fire kills the disease still vital inside the dead carcass as well. Cremation also sends the astral body into the astral plane much quicker than that of the burial of what remains.

What happens to the invisible elements that formed the mind, the emotions, the soul, the astral body? Dissolution of the Astral body occurs through cycles of reincarnation. The soul's break from the karmic emotional body is a gradual process through the law of attraction.

The harmonizing of a disordered impulse within the physical state ascends the elemental ray from the astral body back to the correlating universal element making up the celestial. Human Beings are the only form that hold the rare ability to repair disorder above within the heavens. Thus, the damaged soul purifies itself by removing the desire impulses of the astral plane from its body. Finally, the soul reaches home.

So remember, in order to fix within, start with what you feed it, both in thought and food. Food becomes poison for the lower senses, as nourishment is found in toxic preservatives bound for the intestines, the great storage unit of the toxins. Henceforth, if you have a quarter acre you can still plant or enrich some stuff. You can grow some food, you can enrich the soil. You can even enrich your soul by reading a good book under a beautiful tree!

I will close in the words of Rudolf Steiner, "Anything raised above the normal level for that locale will show a particular tendency to life, a propensity to become permeated with etheric vitality."

[i] The Seven Rays of Life, Alice A. Bailey

Dust

Thomas Medonis

In the beginning God created the heaven and the earth.

And the earth was without form and void, and darkness was upon the face of the deep. And the Spirit of God was moved upon the face of the waters.

-Genesis I: 1-2 King James Version

What if the energy that forms celestial heaven, and the moving energy that keeps earth's motion, is present and active within us? What if this system within is not nearly working at full capability? According to authors' Mantak and Maneewan Chia, there is a "Microcosmic Orbit" within all of us. It is a system within our body that mirrors the Macrocosmic Orbit of our universe. There are two internal energy channels in the human body that need the simple movement of your very own tongue to link these two systems to form the fully functioning "microcosmic orbit" of the human body. The ascending channel runs up the spine ending at the roof of the mouth. The descending channel starts its decent at the tip of the tongue and then down to the lower reproductive organs. Thus, simply pressing the tip of your tongue to the deeper part of the roof of your mouth creates a unified physical being. Your energy is flowing, literally. Nevertheless, there probably are some serious energy blockages in all of our adult bodies. Illness and pain are all a result of an energy blockage.

    Even as physical beings, our flesh, organs, senses, and glands are still all the creation of the same cosmic dust that spreads throughout the primal emptiness.

It doesn't feel that way, but truly the source of all of our emotions, our pains, our love is a primordial void. Yes, the purest refined energy, the process of the universe, can be portrayed as a constantly spiraling circle bearing the fruit of material and spirit. This dust, comprised of galactic waves and particles, that forms the planets and stars, is the same energetic force that spirals into us!

As we wrinkle, lose sight, gain weight, let's stop for a second and realize, we can stop this degradation. The microcosmic must align with the macrocosmic. The earth's stable motion is not hindered in it's 365 day orbit around the sun. The four seasons will commence as sure as the earth continues its harmonious motion. Humans, on the other hand, are very inconsistent when it comes to a natural harmony. Our balance is off even though we are divine dust. The problem is we cannot unite the dust of the cosmos absorbed through our heads, with the vibration of the earth that enters through the soles of our feet. If at all we can unite the two great energy receptors of the cosmos and earth, there is an area within everyone that can become the purest refined energy that is also found in the primal void. Thus we have the power to absorb the original source of creation through extending our consciousness outward to draw in a particular magnifying energy. As they say "As above, so below", the external energies, the movements of the universe, are truly our internal energies too! The alignment into one constant orbit of internal motion makes for a healthy and strong life force.

We haven't been properly educated. Food is broken down galactic dust. We are led to believe the food we put in our body is more important to our health than the thoughts and energetic practices we feed our body. The arousing energy of the universe is alive in everything- wind, breath, water, blood, etc. This cosmic dust can not be created or destroyed, it simply transforms into temporary manifestations. Nothing is permanent, except for the movement of the universe, which is the same primal source for our life force. And this same force responsible for the motion of the planets and stars, and the radiation from the sun, is responsible for our thought and emotional patterns.

When condensed , Chi [Dust] becomes a living being; when dispersed, it is the substratum [basis] of change. - Zhang Tsai (1020-1077 A.D.)

       Will, also known as intention, is imperative to support a functioning internal microcosmic orbit. Intent is the governing state of the body. Without control of the internal life force there will be no stable cosmic connection or strong health. We must truly move our thoughts away from the desires that remove the intention to return to our true nature. Ironically, when we stop focusing our intentions on empty cravings, and we turn our intention to the energy of the sun, moon and stars, we become superheroes that can transform those great sources of energy into power-up's for our own life force. As one improves the circulation of the microcosmic orbit, energy deficiency is resolved.

Health all starts will the will! If the will is weak, the body will be weak. If the will is distracted by enormous amounts of external influences, then there will be no microcosmic orbit. Just as our sexual reproductive energy diminishes following a moment of love, our divine creative dust diminishes. This, however, is not a bad thing as we must become internal alchemist with the energies we feel. To cycle all the energies felt through the microcosmic orbit is to perform alchemy. A strong life force has full control of its sexual energy, as it is all part of one universal system. Is cosmic dust as important as oxygen for human survival? Are they the same thing?

Tip of the tongue on the deepest spot on the roof of your mouth, along with the quieting of the mind, is the beginning of your microcosmic orbit! Yes, external sources take away our life force, however, our bodies can receive and transmute the life force of other "dust" beings. The dust has created everything! Thus, everything in existence has a tremendous impact on our life force. The electromagnetic field of the earth and the moon, for example, draw in galactic dust from billions of stars and planets. The earth's vibration, the sun's rays, sound frequency, all impact our life force. Most importantly, we must let the energy flow…

Further Reading:

Awaken Healing Light of the Tao, Healing Tao Books, Mantak Chia and Maneewan Chia, Huntington, New York, 1993

Down with Disease

Thomas Medonis

"Nature has invented death in order to have much life" - Goethe

To understand disease we must first begin with an admission. Physical energy doesn't exist. Our bodies energy is formed through interactions between planetary energy, warmth, electricity, and magnetism. Thus, we are activated by the laws of nature- a glorious universal harmony that can't be duplicated. The universal mind can however be perceived by our EGO.

We are all formed differently into matter by this universal harmony. All minerals, plants, humans, animals, are shaped through patterns replicating primordial elements. Man, unfortunately, alters nature's eternal echoes during physical evolution. We have the wonderful power of individualizing natural phenomena. Smells, sounds, linen, all stir our EGO. Ironically all the sensations are part of the Universal Mind and it is our EGO that personifies universal elements. The only occurrence when the Universal Mind and the Individual Mind are one and the same is when we are sleeping. This is why we truly get fatigued. Both Universal and Individual Mind's ascend to the higher plane during bedtime. They rejoin the unaltered universal elements. The EGO briefly is home and will return with the next evening.

Awake, grounded on Earth, unfortunately, is when loss of childhood flexibility slowly occurs, while churning and hardening into natural concrete. Yes, the universal harmonious nature is clearly present while we are awake. The EGO quickly finds it through external expression.

Humans hold the rare ability to both ground and form the natural harmony. Yet, this process is quite draining on our vital energies. Human, as earth, evolves, adapts, and changes through time immemorial. In time, the possibility, to embrace the spiritual quality in every living being will evolve. The necessity for the mind to be in a sleep-like state allows for the unification of the forming earthly EGO with the emotional cosmic forces. This is the higher world that has no visibility within our lowest material plane. The EGO's attraction to universal energies display's its means of sustenance. Awoke EGO "food" is magnetized in just as our Earth's balance depends on the universal nature.

Gravity is a prime example of how our great planet magnetizes in undefinable forces through mountain peaks and forests. Gravity, as the movement towards the Earth, is of a different strength in different locations on our home planet. Man, also has such powers of balancing energy. Energetic sensation/perceptions of man first begin as imperceptible rays of vibratory light. This originating force existing in the Universal Mind materializes within a central point- THE EGO. This focal point leads to endless unfathomable separate sensations within the Individual Mind. This point is the only entity of mind in human that all sensations can like to. Thus, the more our ego focus' on earthly desires the greater the natural harmony decreases.

To further physical fatigue, new experience and multiple affairs combine to drain our energy. All that is new to the ego is tiresome or otherwise perceived as

the death/decaying thought principle. It is
in the best interest of our self-
preservation to begin to connect with the
natural harmony within all animate
beings. But, first, most importantly, we
must find the endless harmony in-tune
within our own bodies.

When we begin to connect with memory
photos we begin to travel further with our
soul. On the other hand, our memories
become so bulky by new strange
impressions that the EGO loses the
knowledge of the universal nature, which
is relayed mentally through repeated
memories and emotions. These
continuous repetitious thoughts compile
physical obscurities over time- otherwise
known as illness. Lingering thoughts on
the same matter is a clear indication that
the energetic balance is off. But, too, we
must understand that life started through

the death/decay breakdown process. Is this the reason so many suffer memory disease? Maybe a bad memory isn't even a disease! What if the EGO just couldn't process all the memories/sensations/perceptions occurring. Do memories die?

A solution for memory improvement may simply be found in a fond memory of childhood, or a sore feeling about your first fight never resolved. This simple reflection brings all senses under the rule of EGO. Now we must learn to separate from the material entity and rejoin the all-pervading spiritual plane. The feeling of anger, for instance, is a clear sign of a spiritual weakness. Love, on the other hand, is the great force for both human communication and healing. Growth and health exist when every is n'sync and involuntarily reacting at the right place at the right time. Conversely, loss of vibratory timing leads to the build up of toxins and illness. Thus, the ability must be found within to use these energetic rays manipulating the Universal Mind to our advantage, because they are the "Lifeline" to every living mind. Without the rays colluding within our universe's vastness there would be no growth, no attachment, no form, no animation. We as humans are simply a vehicle of the universal nature, we produce it in our offspring, in our gestures, in our flowers. Down with EGO does not have to mean down with disease. Always be awoke in the HOLY SPIRIT!

THE SPARK

Thomas Medonis

To think the soul is hidden in a vast roller-coaster of bile and gunk is a bit of lunacy. The divine mind's connection to man is a microscopic spot just around the belly button. Our amazing sense perception actually was much more profound when the umbilical chord was connected in utero. Our physical construction forms through this magical connection to the Etheric powers throughout the cosmos. Each individual is truly working to create their own manifestation of this spark. All dimensional planes need to be grounded on this spark to exist. Yet, all planes are not visible and become a bit cluttered if over emphasis on one plane is a consistent mental state. So what the hell do intestines have to do with all this?

The spark is the initial force that first breaks down food. Human waste is not only found in fecal matter. Hair, nails, sweat, blood, poop, pee, all are different avenues for energy breakdown. A very similar freeway exists within the Atmosphere. The Etheric elements are the energy you can't see. Oh yes there are great forces we can't grasp or see, but we sure can feel them. How is that so? Is the decomposing of spirits what truly keeps Earth afloat and humans grounded?

Vibratory frequency is the bridge that turns solid material into energy. Is this process, first begun in the spark, able to be altered? Of course! To truly breakdown waste we must sit still and welcome the universal rhythm pumping energy through us on so many different planes. Welcome it! share your gratitude with the stillness. Love it!

All of this first started with the spark!

How do you find this spark?

What does the spark feel like?

A cosmic rainbow?

What the hell kind of hippy are you?

The spark is the fuel for all Etheric
planes and elements. It is found deep
within the manifestation. Dimensional
planes are what we mentally
broadcast as our reality. Internally,
the physical and mental planes meet
in the Enteric Nervous System. This
network runs through the entire
digestive tract. From the esophagus,
through the stomach and intestines,
down to the anus, the Enteric System
connects all nerves, neurons, and
neurotransmitters. They call this the
Gut-Brain, as the nervous system
regulates the speed of digestion.

However, all of this would cease to exist as soon as the spark dies. This divine spark creates and manifests all of our feelings, emotions, and senses. These feelings felt in our nervous system are felt just as intense in our intestines. Which promotes which? A great first step to identify our mental and physical state is to meditate and get the mind n'sync with the universal formula- a formula in which our bodies engage in every moment. The only other advice this author could share on strengthening the divine spark would be to keep your colon clean!

The Perceptive Stamp

Thomas Medonis

The perceptive stamp of planetary energy force is the blueprint of universal consciousness. Ironically, the force able to imagine prophetic words and create structures is most absent from the normal everyday human. Yes, on the other hand, the philosophy of this force 'of the utmost divine will power' is held in every religion and practice. The definition of this power is where the raw is synthesized.

As a writer of many years and experiences, it is of the utmost importance to use my words as symbols for expression. Writing is a means to carry the spirit home to the soul. Sadly, our media apparatus isn't geared to express soulfulness. Media production stirs about the constant fantasies that tend to draw near our lower desires. Thus, far away from view is the highest

vibrational form of consciousness-
Universal Consciousness! In fact, it
dismays myself to speak from the ego,
but nepotism and neuroticism have taken
up all the leverage for success. Could
such flaws be the result from the
downgrading of divine spiritual media
capital? There are very few avenues
open toward innovative spiritual
evolution. Are we to remain in a fixed
contemporary conduct that parallels that
of delinquent teens?

What is lacking?

Are we looking too far away for an
answer?

Why is the messiah presented the way
he is?

Why do we celebrate gold, fame, and value so highly?

What if our mind's image of perfection is actually the force able to form gold?

The mind's purest form is one and the same as the footprint of a radiant male or female.

Is each religion's savior the likeness to the creative force?

Is our Messiah the structure of the individual universal creating force?

Well, I believe we are all forms of the divine creative force.

For me, the force can be found when we discover what is missing from ourselves within. It is our task to create and house the same Universal Consciousness as all the savior's through time immemorial. What if it was as simple as discovering the divine feminine in males, and the divine male in women? The missing ying to the yang, and yang to the ying. The force most absent in our lives is the same force we must channel in to become truly balanced. Divinity is the accumulation of everything we are not.

Please never forget, the divine feminine or divine male are just as flashes of lightning aside internal seismic thunder. They will never be one and the same. To understand a perfect storm we must view it from afar. An invisible force is always beside us, overlooking, just as we are all illuminated by the moon's light. Our divine better half is a sweet tenderness impossible to duplicate. Well, the closest we can get is through the memory of a mom's presence or of a father's hug. This thought force disappears just as a lightning bolt in the sky, but it is forever present in all of us. A simple thought of our parents brings about the primordial male-female divine creative force in all!

Septenary

Thomas
Medonis

Is it an organ? I don't think so. Is there any way to explore or examine a Chakra? I don't think so.

What if our Chakra system was somehow working in coordination with the stages of the moon?

Rather than how we view the organs as physical examples forming through the production of universal forces, Chakras are mental structures. It has been said that the human chakra system is septenary in nature.

Our heart is considered the radiant central Chakra for the physical body, just as the sun fuels our solar system. Below the heart center are the three inferior chakras, and above the heart are the three superior chakras. Yes, our body is a solar system. Actually, the chakras are the mind's organs. Seven nerve centers in the brain parallel the seven nerve centers on the spine. However, chakras can only be explored through relaxing, withdrawing, and perceiving within.

The spine, or the great link, is considered the great rod that connects all seven chakras with a force that rises out of the head. The three lower chakras, Mars, Mercury, and Jupiter, and the upper three chakras, Saturn, sun, and moon, are all connected to the same spinning axis. The constant motion of pure love fuels this linkage system all because of the hearts, Venus', energetic purpose. This is why we breathe.

I think of rocks or beads to represent chakras, as the one spinal link weaves through all our energetic centers. These rocks located on the spine serve as the individualized nerve centers. These chakras are where certain Etheric Energy enters and circulates into the physical structure. The Chakras (nervous system centers) weave nervous energy into physical manifestation. The nerves mutate into a language with the lymphatic system. Thus, it may come as a surprise, but I am here to write that our Chakras are usually moving in a false motion-aging our body, some at rapid paces! They are spinning the wrong way. What? How? Why am I still alive?

Imagination, too, is all the result of a nervous energetic system. Think of all the thought energy that runs through your mind in cycles everyday. Obsession upon the same thing over and over is simply insanity. The improper motion of a mental energy center grounds the pure energy and ages the nervous system, ultimately aging the physical body, chakras, many write, are simply wheels that are spinning in different directions. Without some esoteric knowledge we spin in the wrong direction all our life. A deviated chakra's purpose is always a negative frequency produced by preconceived conditioning. Our mind projects the product of our nervous energy into thought forms.

Imagine an image, you've created an object! Yes, a mental image, apart from your pure spacious energy, is spinning the individual chakra in the wrong direction as an image is recorded in the brain. Imagination is simply the mind's manipulation of Etheric Energies. This

stored up energy is a false usage. We
need to return these separate energies
back to their universal septenary state, in
order to work in unison, creating an
equilibrium of vibrational frequency
pumping in harmony with the heart's axis.

How do we change the chakras? We
want them to spin in the correct
direction. Well, MEDITATE! Stepping
out of the physical into the Etheric
Energetic body is a wonderful way to
change incorrect energy usage. The true
purpose of the chakra system is the
achievement of physical illumination
through cosmic consciousness. We
become a glowing network of nerves
when we are open. However, we are so
ddp in individual emotional thought we
are unable to float in the cosmos.
Thoughts are attached vibrational forms,
simply, we design mental symbols in an

invisible psychic house. Never forget, physical phenomena begins as mental energy.

We have the power to take the pure consciousness locked in each chakra and trace all that stored past energy back to original conception. A homecoming! Ultimately, inner peace and equilibrium is the pure essence of consciousness.

Each chakra, through meditation, and proper traditional ritual, will open its lotus petals and reveal each of the individual chakras Deities! Keep in mind, no chakra is the same, spins the same, or has the same amount of lotus petals. For one chakra we must choose compassion over passion, another chakra must open with love over hate, radiance over desire.

The true victory in warfare is the outcome of good versus evil. This battle happens within our own mind. If we have the concentration, will, and heart to consistently work on each chakra, we will be victors! The reward is the most valuable accomplishment possible on this earth- The Restoration of Our Pure Nature!

Thus, the seven waterfalls of nerve energy must return to its perfect nature. While we rest in our heart, recognize the radiance that shines! Though, only possible through identifying the pure energy of the top three chakras, along with the nervous, uncontrollable, pulsating energy of the bottom three chakras. It is the nervous energy that travels in these two different directions. We must eliminate that movement to obtain the restoration within the heart- the force of new life. The cerebral and spine are the avenues where energies drive to their home chakra. Interestingly, the etheric energy that is linked to all becomes the physical only through a magnetic field and force. This magnetic force connects our etheric body with our physical body.

Recognition of the pure energy that comprises the etheric body is all possible through the release of our individual mind. It is found inside the heart, it is the golden link. The seat of goodness over illusion.

As the chakras are always spinning our mind is always in motion. We have the power to alter the ego into the infinite pure essence. Every force that is bound must be liberated at some point. The drive of the will must empower each individual to break through the roadblock and get back home.

Some say the arrival of pure consciousness in each chakra reflects God's acceptance. We are accepted into the kingdom when the spirit of light and dark have made peace. Our heart center, once open, with its twelve petals, releases our bondage. We are now able to live within our heart that keeps our hopes and beliefs pure and loving. A new mind is a victory for our soul, but first, we must learn to sit in the stable universal septenary design.

Universal Cleaning Cycle Challenge

Thomas Medonis

Imagine if you will that the unparalleled framework of the human species is identical to our macrocosmic universe. What if our body holds seasonal cycles within us just as the earth? Maybe, illness, rather than a disparaging disposition is the greatest cleansing detox we could ever experience.

Are we supposed to naturally get the flu bug every year and actually use our natural immunity to fight the illness? Cleaning all impurity. Our body's condition during ailment is a great indication of the weaknesses in certain locations. Within, is a system that uses illness to highlight where deviation from the norm actually becomes the norm.

The universal cleansing cycle makes clear our physical problems. Medication, however, is the great manipulator of the universal force. Consequently, through consistent synthetic use, the nervous system, organs, blood, etc., become altered from the natural cyclical state. It is within the universal design that our answers for health will be found, just as a wound heals itself. The cycle of the universe is our nature. Death and disease are simply the universe's cycle visible in its physical state. With death, however, brings about rebirth. Thus, a bad flu should symbolize it is time to recalibrate your deviated energy centers. The challenge is to change!

The Lost
Dance

Thomas
Medonis

Ceremony of the purest energy in a moment of shared love by a community to further the commitment to carry on- is why we should dance. In unison with the universe, inside this dance all energies are alive- ridicule, danger, anger, love. Most dominant in ancient indigenous ceremony is the force to carry the stories of these energy channels on to younger generations. The many ancient Aztec tribes portrayed many indigenous traditions of dance, universal signs, and symbols. Indigenous tribes ironically shared the same symbol as Christianity- The Cross.

Old tradition, oddly, is now almost completely lost. Few scholars of ancient manuscripts are still alive. Ancient manuscripts made of stone preserving the same root and same beginnings of this Great Earth and Human Species also preserve this great ancient tradition of dance. Mainstream education is not in accord with indigenous historians. Corporate Education for some reason doesn't want to understand the old form.

To begin, Ceremonial Dance is based on its region and traditions. Maybe the tribal character is not what education wants. Scholars have argued that indigenous manners lead to ignorance and an uncivilized life. On the contrary, a specific region tells a great story of not only the people's development but the nature of the land itself- not a one world view. The manifestation of each tribe's ceremony is as much due to the region as to its peoples.

All life's movement and energy was displayed in the indigenous people's cross, while the sun was the great energetic source of origin. Pure Solar Essence is Pure Solar Essence. What exists in the great Sun that energizes our entire planet exists in our sons, daughters, and ourselves. Old traditions tell of the sun as the father and earth the mother. There, long ago, was a different consciousness.

An understanding that the planets, the moon, and the stars' energies are all in constant dependence of the sun was etched in ancient stone. Yet, this philosophy seems more like science. A movement of all our body parts- ten toes, ten fingers- moving in harmony with the universe's energies were what told the ancient law that governed the primordials. This understanding portrayed in dance displayed that both birth and death are held at the same esteem. One could not exist without the other. The duality of positive and negative, masculine and feminine, are the very energies that create life. If there is no masculine there is no creation, if there is no feminine there is no creation. For life to continue, it needs death. Life transforms into death, death transforms into life. The two halves make a whole.

The Ancient Elders held the knowledge that death was but a step, a transition, as it was the transformation of energy. Fallen ancestors would be celebrated toward the sun of the dead, as those dancing knew that those no longer with flesh still continued the living energies in another form.

Ancient books had existed and still to this day exist based on the destiny of a newborn. I can easily find a couple books written on the traits of someone born on every day of the year. More passionately felt in ancient tradition was the necessity to fulfill one's written destiny. Everyone has their own life's journey, and the ancients knew that the accomplishment of this mission was to the benefit of the ceremony. Obeying the harmonious laws of the universe was the only way through and these human struggles were manifested in dance. Thus, one would be well versed in the universe if educated in ancient dance theory. Our place of origin transforms through spirituality into a material being with memories and emotions.

We must never forget that the spirit of the universe, holding everything together, is inside of us. And there is both light and dark. After light there is dark, after dark there is light. In life there is death, and in death there is life. One cell has to die to reproduce into two. Think of the beginning of a human. The sperm and egg unite. Male energy and female energy combine and the egg dies. Yet on the contrary, it reproduces and transforms into a human embryo! As we are developing and growing our cells are also dying. After eighty years on this planet they say cells don't die anymore. They live on. This is when we prepare to die. Thus life depends on death, death depends on life.

Unfortunately, all this ancient wisdom was eliminated as foriegn settlers' eliminated any great Ceremonial Dance. These beautiful powerful moments in time would sadly become defined as acts of a savage. A great culture of spiritual understandings would become lost.

Lost was the understanding of the twenty universal channels felt through the twenty fingers and toes. The particular influence of energies in each day could be read. Colors were also greatly used to define the movement and transformation of energies. Red would share masculine heat, while blue would portray feminine calm. The ancient knowledge also told of the thirteen articulations of the human. These thirteen main arteries are what connects us with the universal forces. Furthermore, these ancients knew the best tool for measuring the universe was the human body. From within, we must discover the movement of life.

Indigenous tribes actually used the cross to teach the concept of life. The cross represented the four directions, the four seasons- the movement of the universe around the sun. The cross was life and death. Death is transition, movement is life, thus death is life. We must never forget even as Mother Earth is always transforming, the feminine energy is still governed by the moon. Why do we elect those to create laws, when in actuality, if we are properly educated in universal law, our conduct would mirror that of the heavens. Laws of transformation and change should always take precedent.

Surprisingly, one thing changing and always dying is our great sun. The truth of our human energy is found inside the sun. Elders described the inside of the sun as some type of a form or figure, holding an appearance similar to that of a skull. This skull represents death and transformation. The sun is dying, but the transformation and movement into life is happening in the center nucleus.

Again, why is the sun dying? Well, as it dies it gives us back all its new energy. From this dying sun comes all the energy for the solar system. We came from above, died below, and have to move and transform to reach up above again.

We must never forget that the dance is sacrificial. Sacred songs, sacred drum beats, sacred dances are all sacrifices to other earthlings' well-being. The law of duality- positive and negative, masculine and feminine.

The ancients knew the song of creation. Sounds displaying the moving frequencies within the universe were brought together through the harmony of drum and rattle. Oh, the harmony of the universe, this is why we DANCE! All forms of conduct is a part of the great dance. Though, peace and justice will only arrive when the law of universal consciousness is held by all!

Maldek

Thomas
Medonis

We live in a day where a voice sharing an alternative idea leads to multiple negative labels. One label would most certainly be that of lunacy if a citizen of law and order was to disagree with criminal corruption of the "Elites". Well, I grasp for all trophies.

Just imagine, not too hard, that the greatest threat to human being' living existence is the very "will" inside a human being. This force has already destroyed an earth-like planet, Maldek, as well as multiple civilizations, Lemuria and Atlantis. Here we are, all of us humans, at a collective boiling point. A planet's well-being, its very own living existence, all depends on its populace!

Yes, we are that powerful. Material is the gross form of mind. Ying-Yang, good-bad, all material is created for better or worse. What if the most holy of beings reside on other planets based on vibratory frequency? Lunacy I tell you. Our minds are currently spiritually unable to interpret these levels of energetic vibration. What if this cosmic consciousness travels through consciousness rather than time and space?

Are we capable of reaching a trance like state emulating a planets vibratory rhythm? Are these powers located on different energy centers on the physical body? If the universal rhythm has an effect on our whole, do we have an effect on our whole, do we have an effect on the rhythm? This vibratory rhythm holds the space I define as the "Etheric Ocean", uniting all the collective energy waves flying through the air. Both positive and negative impulses are found in the sky, as well as our mind. As the mind radiates thoughts, its energy radiation is morphed.

Radiation in its most subtle form is still an etheric energy. Thus, positive/negative charges can form a chain reaction when combined with an attracting force. The manifestation of an atomic chain reaction is the most physical devastating manifestation possible on earth.

No, I don't want to think about our planet's destruction by our very own 'minds' and 'will'. To avoid this agony I bring my mind to what would term a "negative" type of trance- "Thinking," snap of anger, "empty pitcher". We must not think. The greatest intelligences are available at all times. We are the only one's capable to mess up the divine will. Etheric radiation will attract to positive/negative energy, and build upon this. This may be the fact why many argue that anyone has super-natural powers. Yes, we can all perform scientific healing procedures on others through the psychic centers sitting in the palms of our hands. For this to be possible, we must first raise our psychic current from the point of our darkest desires and acts, and guide it to the chakra of the heavens to activate new intelligences. Strangely, these intelligences are only found through prolonged concentration within etheric channels (hollow beams), which are the bridges of these thought transmissions.

Another trance state my mind is able to sit in and create occurs when myself no longer exists. My rhythm becomes that of a subjective mental radiation- a mental concept. More or less, a transmission within the mind attracts thought impulses radiating a magnetic Etheric wave frequency. This could be considered a positive mind trance as theming focuses on the individual psychic energy currents, slowly growing an ability to live within and translate these energy impulses.

We all will reach these frequencies, but at different stages of development and lifetimes. The path of evolution is not only travelled on by our physical bodies, but it is our soul that never leaves the trail of Divine Will. So, we have this amazing eternal loving soul, yet, that as Earth Creatures is our last concern. Why do we always put the least important in front of the most important? We already, all of us, have within us, this amazing cosmic consciousness. A mental state beyond enlightenment, this consciousness is a state when individual mind ceases. All that exists is the "oneness" of eternity.

The Etheric Ocean pervades everything, not only on earth, but universally. The ability to join eternal rest is the last stage in order for an individual's reincarnations to stop forever. The minds rise in positive Etheric frequency is the key for freedom of rebirth. Thus, we must celebrate all living beings including our mind, but most importantly, though, we must celebrate the Earth! Earth has the most glorious light radiation available to all her children. Her manifestations are available every second of every day. This light must be felt in our minds. It must be the force that dawn's the new age. However, keep in mind, synthesizing earth's vibratory rhythm disrupts the cosmic essence in all natural material.

I pray one day a group of men of "Divine Will" will initiate a new age of thought and conduct on earth, which will no doubt bring discomfort to those living corrupt untruthful lives. The true nature has been withheld for too long! Use karma as the greatest tool available. Learn from your karmic state rather than repeat it. Things will repeat if we don't learn the true past.

Millions of years ago a small planet made an orbit between Mars and Jupiter. Maldek was similar in size to Earth. It was a lush green planet where destruction first began to evolve when a minute disease that called the mind home began to spread. Unfortunately as the lust for power spread so rapidly and powerfully, Maldek was soon destroyed through multiple forms of atomic energy. The exploded remnants of Maldek formed the asteroid belt- cold spinning rock. This self-sustaining planet was destroyed by its own people! Earth civilizations of Lemuria and Atlantis held the same fate. Yes, the asteroid belt is formed of remnants of a planet destroyed by its own residents, the human race.

A people so civilized created technology so powerful to destroy an entire planet. Planet Maldek exploded eighteen million years ago. However, the human race of Maldek was so in tune with cosmic intelligences that they kept form through consciousness and descended through

the Etheric Ocean, reaching the lone
residents of Earth, the Adamic Man.
Surprisingly, of all the planets, the only
one accepting those dark forces of
Maldek was Earth.

Earth was the lone planet welcoming a
citizenry that watched without questioning
the dire consequences of limitless
technology and power. Spirit does not
empower technology, our 'will' does. But
spirit is strong in us, because the earth is
able to use us as a medium to ground
this amazing indefinable force! May we
all one day work together with the Earth,
just as compassionate as our mother has
been with us, and combine spiritual
service with the available technology to
improve, enhance, and payback our
loving mother!

Allopathic

Vs.

Homeopathic

Thomas Medonis

If I told you our very own government funds research on Bio-Weapons, would you be concerned? Or, would you respond, "Huh, what the heck is that?"

I've heard of Geo-Engineering by our government. Just look up and you will see chemtrails being sprayed throughout the skies by unmanned drones. I suppose the use of synthetic man-made aerosols has many purposes: control of the weather, nano-particle surveillance, spreading bio-weapons, blocking sunlight, etc.

"Drones" and "exercises" are very frightening terms when used by the military industrial complex through Department of Defense (D.O.D.) funding. The M2SR Virus Vaccine, which focuses on the M2 protein, granted Professor Kawaoka a $ 14.4 million dollar State Department Contract, through University of Wisconsin. Bio-Tech labs at University of Wisconsin are clear evidence that our money is truly being spent on nefarious purposes, rather than our very own health and healing.

Schools unfortunately have been taken over. Education is where healthcare and medicine have become manipulated for monetary purpose rather than natural healing. In the 1800's American's had options. There was Allopathic medicine and Homeopathic medicine. Allopathic medicine is cutting-edge science, medicine, and surgery- modern medical system. Homeopathic medicine relies on natural herbs, and naturalistic practices that stimulate the individual body's natural immune system- old traditional medicine.

In this pre-planned multi-generational enhancement of medical technology one thing was overlooked- HEALING! Thus, John D. Rockefeller, through The Rockefeller Foundation has shaped

American medicine through our educational process. The Rockefeller Foundation placed multiple board members on every single school's 'board of directors', all in order for money to be spent properly. And was it spent! For a large hospital system to work with all new radiology departments, operational equipment, and experimental drugs, it needed people trained to spend and use all resources.

The sneaky thing the American Medical Association

(AMA) did when it was founded in 1847 was to prohibit a license to any homeopathic physician, still in effect to this day. Thus doctors became more educated on synthetic drugs rather than natural remedies. In 1910, the investigation on the quality of medical education in all 161 medical schools that existed was conducted by Abraham Flexner in "The Flexner Report". As a result, credibility and funding for nearly all schools using non-drug based medicine was removed. As this book-length landmark report was sponsored through the Carnegie Foundation, "The Flexner Report" completely changed the framework of medicine. This coup against natural medicine formed the necessity for the accreditation of hospitals. Flexnor, hired and paid for by Rockefeller and Carnegie (AMA), was not even a doctor, he was simply on the staff of the Carnegie Foundation for the advancement of "Teaching".

Through the removal of "teaching" natural medicine, and the advancement of technological medicine, people could no longer afford such extravagant equipment and procedures. Insurance would thus become a necessary social program.

With the American League of Municipalities (Small towns) and the American Association of State Government (State Legislature) being under the oversight and guidance of the

Rockefeller Foundation, the legislature became a tool to draft new measures in order to develop hospitals and doctors. Doctors and hospitals were only licensed by the legislature, which proves the fact that only the Rockefeller Foundation could approve a medical license. Doctors are employees of the government, and actually, the AMA has brought charges against doctors curing people. Consequently, the Rockefeller Foundation has control of every drug manufacturer in the world.

The addition of modern medicine with corporate capitalists equates to a manipulated healthcare system that doesn't provide healing. We have been duped! Obamacare is a fraud in order to eliminate wealth. Private insurers, lobbyists, bribed public servants, educational administrators, are all co-conspirators in this ponzi scheme to diminish your wealth and health. How much do public servants really receive from private healthcare?

Our free god-given natural healing powers have been hijacked! The Eugenic Depopulation Cartel rules every aspect of our lives. In the 1990's multiple countries were unknowingly injected with anti-fertility vaccines! In India fertility control agents were administered, as the Rockefeller Foundation knows no limit to pain. Planned Parenthood and The

Population Council are funded under grants from the Rockefeller Foundation, all in order to remove whatsoever DNA they want removed from the genetic human make-up.

In this day of "$1,000 pills" and "Vaccine prevention", we are prohibited from letting universal nature take part in our health, even as creatures formed through the Earth. Yet, that is the solution. Why are we not curing anything with simple cheap solutions? Monetary control is the

Imperial way. And it was, it is, and it will be our way until we change being healed by the greedy.

Pole Star

Thomas Medonis

If dark matter is 96% of the universe, is this why light is so important?

Light frequency is the new healing. How?

To understand the new medicine, we must view our emotions and feelings in terms of colors and energy. Anger and fear stir our dark burgundy energy. While, unconditional love produces violet light energy. And yes, this violet light pervades everything and is omnipresent in every form and object. Where does this colored energy derive from?

Well, there is an energy axis within our body that unites with the North Star. The North Star or "Pole Star" is our soul's gateway to heaven. And just as souls move and the earth moves, the designation of the Pole Star gradually changes over time. The violet light emanates from this North Star focal point. Thus, the spirit begins a new journey upon the time of death. Hopefully, it is a brisk quick trip back to the source of unconditional love.

Quite simply, Polaris, or also known as North Star or Pole Star, is the the center star of its star field. The Pole Star is so important because the axis of Earth is pointed nearly directly at it. Throughout the night, Polaris does not rise or set, but remains still in the same location above the northern horizon all year. Consequently, the other stars circle around it.

Moreover, Polaris is around 50 times the size of our sun. The sun's estimated diameter is around 44 million miles (70 million kilometers), and a radius of about 22 million miles (35 million kilometers). According to experts, the North Star is slowly shrinking, and data reveals that the focal point in the northern sky is releasing an Earth's mass worth of gas each year.

The Pole Star seems dim to us because it is so far away from Earth. However, conversely, the star is a giant— a yellow supergiant in a short-lived stage before the star inflates into a red supergiant. Astronomers make the prediction that the Pole Star will shed off its outer shell, which will force the helium on the inside to start burning. Consequently, the heavier elements then will burn until it is primarily all iron. After nearly another million years or so, the core will explode, in which a supernova will form.

Polaris, designated α Ursae Minoris, is the brightest star of the constellation Ursa Minor. It is very close to the north celestial pole, making it the current northern pole star. The revised Hipparcos parallax gives a distance to Polaris of about 433 light-years away, while calculations by some other methods derive distances up to 35% closer.

Polaris is a triple star system, composed of the primary star, Polaris Aa (a yellow supergiant), in orbit with a smaller companion (Polaris Ab); the pair in orbit with Polaris B (August 1779 by William Herschel). (Wikipedia)

To rejoin Polaris, the soul's energy departs from the physical through a point on the top of the head, known as "The Crown". This tip top point in our body welcomes in Polaris's heavenly energy at birth (unconditional love), and yet, also is the release point of our remaining energy at death.

If we are able to bring awareness into the heavenly energy frequency, we are able to skip many trials for our soul after death. Even alive, if you can stay in a state of unconditional love 24/7, then your body will not age. Our thoughts are magical as they turn pure energy into decaying matter. Thus, we must practice and meditate in coordination with the universal forces and motions.

In the head, the Hypothalamus Gland is also found. "The hypothalamus is involved in different daily activities like eating or drinking, in the control of the body's temperature and energy maintenance, and in the process of memorizing and in stress control. It also modulates the endocrine system through its connections with the pituitary gland." (Intechopen.com)

Simplified, the Hypothalamus Gland is the pathway for our vibrant red energy to connect with the red vibrant energy the Big Dipper produces. The red vibrant vital energy of the Big Dipper, also the same energy as the vitality of our life force, is found within ourselves too! Aside from blood, where in our bodies is this red energy first absorbed?

The area of the brain where the Hypothalamus, Pineal, and Pituitary glands are found is defined as the crystal room. This glandular unit has the ability to create a golden light body. When unified with awareness in pure energy the physical body transforms into a golden light form.

The purification of our energy through our internal crystals unlocks our true pure energetic spirit. The frequency of our golden light body is universally designed to leave the decaying physical body. Focus on the eternal nature of unconditional love and we will forever be free! Never forget, compassion is the greatest form of universal nature. It is the key to heaven.